Eat To Overcome your Diet

Nourishing Your Body, Mind, and Soul for Lasting Well-Being

Dr John T. Grover

Copyright

Copyright © Dr John T. Grover 2024. All rights reserved. Before this document is duplicated or reproduced in any manner, the publisher's consent must be gained. Therefore, the contents within can neither be stored electronically, transferred, nor kept in a database. Neither in Part nor full can the document be copied, scanned, faxed, or retained without approval from the publisher or creator.

Table of content

Eat to overcome your diet

Dedication

To all those on a journey of self-discovery through the intricate world of nutrition, this book is dedicated to you. May "Eat to Overcome Your Diet" serve as a compass, guiding you through the maze of dietary choices, fostering a healthier relationship with food, and empowering you to overcome the challenges on your path to well-being. Your commitment to embracing a nourishing lifestyle inspires this dedication, as together we navigate the delicious intersection of health and happiness.

From a sincere heart

Dr John T. Grover

Author Bio

Dr. John T. Grover is a distinguished author whose expertise transcends boundaries, blending his profound knowledge in the field of expertise with a passion for storytelling. With a wealth of experience, he navigates the complexities of specific subjects with a unique narrative flair, making his works both intellectually stimulating and accessible to a diverse audience. Driven by a relentless curiosity, he has authored numerous insightful publications, earning him recognition as a thought leader in relevant industry. His commitment to excellence in both academia and literature makes Dr. Grover a compelling voice in the literary landscape.

Introduction:

Welcome to "Eat to Overcome Your Diet," a journey toward redefining your relationship with food and transcending the limitations of traditional dieting. This book is not a strict set of rules or a one-size-fits-all solution. Instead, it invites you to explore a holistic approach to nourishment—one that considers not only the science behind eating but also the intricate interplay between your mindset, emotions, and overall well-being.

Together, we will unravel the mysteries of nutritional basics, delve into the art of mindful eating, and discover sustainable habits that go beyond mere calorie counting. It's time to shift the focus from restriction to empowerment,

Eat to overcome your diet

from guilt to joy. Through this exploration, you'll learn to build a balanced plate that fuels your body, satisfies your taste buds, and supports your unique journey toward a healthier, happier you.

Join me in this transformative adventure as we navigate the complexities of eating, overcome challenges, and create a lifestyle that celebrates the richness of nourishing foods.

CHAPTER 1

Understanding Your Relationship with Food

Your journey toward a healthier lifestyle begins with a profound understanding of your relationship with food. Beyond the mere act of eating, this relationship is a complex interplay of emotions, habits, and cultural influences. By delving into the layers of this connection, you gain the insights needed to make informed and mindful choices about what, when, and why you eat.

Unraveling Emotional Associations:

Explore the emotional ties you have with food. Are certain foods linked to comfort, stress relief, or celebration? Understanding these associations allows you to navigate emotional eating patterns and build a healthier, more conscious connection with the foods you choose.

Identifying Triggers and Patterns:

Examine the triggers that lead to your eating habits. Whether it's stress, boredom, or specific environments, recognizing these patterns empowers you to respond thoughtfully rather than reactively. This self-awareness lays the foundation for breaking free from unhealthy cycles.

Mindful Eating Practices:

Introduce the concept of mindful eating—a practice rooted in being present and fully engaged during meals. By savoring each bite, paying attention to hunger and fullness cues, and appreciating the sensory experience of eating, you cultivate a more mindful relationship with food.

Nurturing a Positive Mindset:
Shift the focus from viewing food as the enemy or a source of guilt to seeing it as a means of nourishment and pleasure. Cultivate a positive mindset that values the role of food in fueling your body, supporting your well-being, and enhancing your overall quality of life.

.The Mindset Shift: Eating to Overcome, Not Restrict

In a world where diets often dictate what we can't eat, it's time for a revolutionary mindset shift—one that centers around eating to

Eat to overcome your diet

overcome, not restrict. Instead of approaching nutrition with a mindset of deprivation, this perspective empowers you to make choices that support your well-being, enhance your vitality, and ultimately lead to a sustainable and fulfilling relationship with food.

Embracing Abundance Over Deprivation:
Turn your attention to what you're receiving instead of what you're giving up. Rather than dwelling on restrictions, celebrate the abundance of nourishing options available. Recognize that making positive food choices is about adding vitality and flavor to your life, not subtracting enjoyment.

Building a Positive Connection with Food:

Reframe the way you perceive food. Instead of categorizing it as "good" or "bad," view it as a source of nourishment that contributes to your overall health. This shift in perspective encourages a positive and compassionate approach to eating, fostering a healthy relationship with food.

Listening to Your Body:

Move away from external rules and restrictions and tune in to your body's signals. By listening to hunger and fullness cues, you empower yourself to make choices aligned with your body's needs. This intuitive approach promotes a sustainable and personalized way of nourishing yourself.

Celebrating Food as Fuel:

View food as more than just a source of pleasure or temptation—acknowledge it as fuel for your body and mind. Recognize the impact different foods have on your energy levels, cognitive function, and overall well-being. This awareness lays the foundation for making choices that support your health goals.

Making Informed Choices:

Equip yourself with knowledge about nutrition without falling into the trap of rigid rules. Understand the nutritional value of foods and how they contribute to your overall health. This knowledge empowers you to make informed choices based on your unique preferences and dietary needs.

Cultivating a Growth Mindset:

Approach your journey with a growth mindset, viewing challenges as opportunities for learning and improvement. Embrace the idea that your relationship with food is dynamic and can evolve positively over time. This mindset shift fosters resilience and adaptability on your path to a healthier lifestyle.

By adopting the mindset of eating to overcome rather than restrict, you pave the way for a sustainable, enjoyable, and transformative approach to nutrition. This shift not only empowers you to make choices that align with your well-being but also fosters a positive and harmonious relationship with the diverse and delicious world of food.

CHAPTER 2

Building a Balanced Plate

Building a balanced plate is essential for maintaining a healthy and well-rounded diet. A balanced plate ensures that you receive a variety of nutrients, vitamins, and minerals, promoting overall well-being and preventing nutritional deficiencies. Here's a guide to help you create a nourishing and balanced plate:

1.Include a Variety of Colorful Vegetables:

Aim to fill half of your plate with a diverse range of colorful vegetables. Different colors indicate various nutrients, so mix it up with

leafy greens, red peppers, carrots, and other vibrant options

2. Add Lean Proteins:

Incorporate lean proteins like chicken, fish, tofu, or legumes. Proteins are essential for immune system function, muscle repair, and general bodily upkeep. Choose grilled, baked, or steamed options to keep it healthy.

3. Whole Grains for Sustained Energy:

Choose whole grains like whole wheat, quinoa, or brown rice. These include fiber, complex carbs, and vital minerals. They help in maintaining steady energy levels and promoting digestive health.

4. Healthy Fats in Moderation:

Add foods like avocados, almonds, and olive oil that are good sources of fat. These fats are important for brain health, hormone production, and the absorption of fat-soluble vitamins.

5. Portion Control: Be mindful of portion sizes. Even healthy foods can contribute to excess calorie intake if portion sizes are too large. To assist with portion control and stop overindulging, use smaller plates.

6. **Reduce the Intake of Processed Foods and Added Sugars:** Cut back on the amount of processed foods and foods high in added sugars. These can contribute to weight gain, inflammation, and various health issues. Choose whole, natural foods whenever possible.

7. Seek Professional Guidance: See a licensed dietitian or nutritionist if you have any special health goals or concerns. They are able to offer tailored guidance according to your particular requirements and way of life. Remember, building a balanced plate is not about strict rules but rather about creating a sustainable and enjoyable way of eating that nourishes your body. It's a foundation for long-term health and wellness.

Portion Control and Serving Sizes

Understanding Portion Control and Serving Sizes for a Healthy Lifestyle:

Maintaining a healthy lifestyle involves more than just choosing nutritious foods; it also requires being mindful of portion control and serving sizes. Proper portion control plays a crucial role in managing weight, preventing overeating, and ensuring that your body receives the right balance of nutrients. Here's a comprehensive guide to help you navigate portion control and serving sizes:

1. What is Portion Control?

Portion control involves managing the amount of food you eat at a single sitting. It's about being aware of how much you're consuming to avoid excess calorie intake. This practice is vital for weight management and overall well-being.

2. The Importance of Serving Sizes

Understanding recommended serving sizes is key to achieving a balanced diet. Serving sizes are standardized measurements that help consumers compare similar foods and make informed choices. They also assist in controlling calorie intake and preventing overconsumption.

3. Read Nutrition Labels:

Nutrition labels on packaged foods provide information about serving sizes and the number of servings per container. Pay attention to these labels to make informed decisions about your food intake. Be mindful of serving sizes, especially if a package contains more than one serving.

4.Choose Nutrient-Dense Foods:

Opt for nutrient-dense foods that provide essential vitamins and minerals without excessive calories. Vegetables, fruits, lean proteins, and whole grains are excellent choices for balanced nutrition.

5. Staying hydrated

Don't overlook liquid calories. Beverages, including sugary drinks and even some seemingly healthy options, can contribute significantly to your daily calorie intake. Choose water, herbal tea, or other low-calorie options to stay hydrated.

6. Avoid Distractions During Meals:

Mindless overeating can result from eating while preoccupied with something else, such watching TV or working. Make an effort to eat without distractions, savoring each bite and paying attention to your body's signals.

7. Practice Moderation, Not Deprivation:

Portion control is not about deprivation but rather moderation. Enjoy your favorite foods in smaller amounts, and savor the flavors. This

Eat to overcome your diet

approach makes healthy eating more sustainable in the long run.

Creating Nutrient-Rich Meals

Crafting Nutrient-Rich Meals for Optimal Health

Building nutrient-rich meals is a cornerstone of maintaining good health and vitality. Nutrient-rich foods provide essential vitamins, minerals, and other compounds that support overall well-being, energy levels, and disease prevention. Here's a guide to help you create meals that are not only delicious but also packed with the nourishment your body needs:

1. Prioritize Whole Foods:

Base your meals around whole, minimally processed foods. Fruits, vegetables, whole grains, lean meats, and good fats are a few of these.

2. Include a Rainbow of Colors:

Include a range of vibrant fruits and vegetables in your diet. Different colors often indicate various phytonutrients and antioxidants. Aim for a diverse palette to ensure a broad spectrum of nutrients.

3. Choose Lean Proteins:

Opt for lean protein sources such as poultry, fish, beans, tofu, and legumes. Immune system performance, muscle repair, and general cellular health all depend on protein. Vary protein sources to ensure a complete range of amino acids.

4. Embrace Whole Grains:

Eat to overcome your diet

Include whole grains like quinoa, brown rice, oats, and whole wheat in your meals. Whole grains provide complex carbohydrates, fiber, and important nutrients, offering sustained energy and promoting digestive health.

5. Don't Fear Healthy Fats:

InAdd foods like avocados, almonds, seeds, and olive oil that are good sources of fat. Healthy fats are vital for brain health, hormone production, and the absorption of fat-soluble vitamins A, D, E, and K.

6.Limit Added Sugars and Salt:

Minimize the consumption of added sugars and excessive salt. Too much sugar and salt can contribute to various health issues. Choose natural sweeteners like honey or maple syrup and use herbs and spices to enhance flavor.

The Importance of Hydration

The Crucial Role of Hydration in Wellness:
Proper hydration is fundamental to maintaining overall health and well-being. Water, often referred to as the elixir of life, plays a vital role in numerous bodily functions, and adequate hydration is essential for optimal physical and mental functioning. Here's a comprehensive look at the importance of hydration and why staying adequately hydrated is crucial for your health:

1. Cellular Function and Nutrient Transport:
-Water is a fundamental component of cells, facilitating various biochemical processes. Adequate hydration ensures efficient nutrient

transport to cells, contributing to optimal cellular function.

2. Temperature Regulation: Sweating is the body's natural cooling mechanism. Staying hydrated helps regulate body temperature, preventing overheating and supporting the body's ability to adapt to different environmental conditions.

3. Cognitive Function: Dehydration can impair cognitive function, affecting concentration, alertness, and short-term memory. Maintaining proper hydration levels is crucial for mental clarity and overall cognitive performance.

4. Joint Lubrication:

Water plays a key role in joint lubrication. Proper hydration helps maintain joint flexibility and reduces the risk of joint-related discomfort or injuries.

5. Digestive Health:

Water is essential for digestion and nutrient absorption. It helps break down food, supports the movement of nutrients through the digestive tract, and prevents constipation by softening stools.

6. Energy Levels:

Dehydration can lead to feelings of fatigue and reduced energy levels. Staying hydrated supports endurance and helps sustain energy throughout physical activities.

7. Kidney Function:

The kidneys rely on an adequate water supply to filter waste and toxins from the blood, producing urine. Proper hydration supports kidney function and helps prevent kidney stones and urinary tract infections.

8. Skin Health: Hydrated skin appears more vibrant and is less prone to dryness and irritation. Water helps maintain skin elasticity, promoting a youthful appearance and supporting the body's natural detoxification processes.

9. Weight Management:

Getting your water intake in before meals will help you feel fuller and cut back on calories overall. Furthermore, maintaining adequate hydration promotes metabolic functions, which help with weight control.

10. Immune System Support:

Water is necessary for the immune system to operate correctly. Hydration helps transport immune cells and antibodies throughout the body, contributing to a robust defense against infections.

12. Prevention of Dehydration-Related Issues:

Chronic dehydration can lead to various health issues, including kidney stones, urinary tract infections, and electrolyte imbalances. Regular, adequate water intake is a simple yet effective preventive measure.

CHAPTER 3

Sustainable Eating Habits for a Healthier Planet and You

In an era where the impact of our choices on the environment is more evident than ever, adopting sustainable eating habits is not only beneficial for the planet but also for our health. Sustainable eating involves making choices that promote environmental conservation, support local communities, and prioritize health. Here's a guide to help you embrace sustainable eating habits:

1. Choose Plant-Based Options:

- Increase the amount of plant-based foods you eat. Plant-based diets generally have a lower environmental footprint compared to diets high in animal products. Opt for fruits, vegetables, legumes, and whole grains to diversify your meals.

2. Support Local and Seasonal Produce:
Choose locally sourced and seasonal produce whenever possible. This not only reduces the carbon footprint associated with transportation but also supports local farmers and promotes agricultural diversity.

3. Minimize Food Waste: Plan your meals, store food carefully, and use leftovers to reduce food waste.. Composting is an excellent way to further reduce waste and contribute to healthier soils.

4. Embrace Sustainable Proteins:

Choose sustainably sourced proteins such as wild-caught fish, pasture-raised poultry, and ethically produced meats. Explore plant-based protein alternatives like tofu, tempeh, and legumes for variety.

7. Choose Sustainable Seafood:

When consuming seafood, opt for sustainably sourced options to support healthy ocean ecosystems. Look for certifications such as MSC (Marine Stewardship Council) to ensure responsible fishing practices.

8. Grow Your Own:

If you can, grow a little garden in your house. Growing your own herbs, fruits, or vegetables can be a rewarding and sustainable way to

Eat to overcome your diet

supplement your diet while reducing reliance on store-bought produce.

9. Educate Yourself:

Stay informed about sustainable food practices and ethical food production. Understanding the impact of your choices empowers you to make informed decisions that align with your values.

Developing Healthy Eating Habits

Nurturing Healthy Eating Habits for a Lifetime of Wellness

Developing healthy eating habits is a transformative journey that goes beyond temporary diets and fads. It involves cultivating a sustainable and nourishing relationship with food, supporting not only physical health but also overall well-being. Here's a comprehensive guide to help you embark on the path of developing and maintaining healthy eating habits:

1.Embrace Whole, Nutrient-Rich Foods:
Prioritize whole foods that are as close to their natural state as possible. Fruits, vegetables, whole grains, lean proteins, and healthy fats provide essential nutrients that support various bodily functions.

2.Mindful Eating Practices:
Practice mindful eating by savoring each bite, paying attention to flavors and textures, and being present during meals. This approach helps you appreciate food and prevents overeating.

3.Balanced Meals:

Eat to overcome your diet

Strive for balanced meals that include a mix of macronutrients. Incorporate carbohydrates, proteins, and healthy fats to ensure a well-rounded and nourishing diet.

4.Diversify Your Plate:

Include a variety of colors on your plate to ensure a broad spectrum of nutrients. Different colors in fruits and vegetables often indicate distinct health benefits.

5. Plan and Prepare Meals:

Plan your meals in advance and prepare them at home whenever possible. This empowers you to make healthier choices and have control over the ingredients in your dishes.

6.Lifelong Learning:

Eat to overcome your diet

View healthy eating as a journey of continuous learning. Explore new recipes, try different cuisines, and remain open to adapting your eating habits based on your evolving understanding of nutrition.

Incorporating Variety into Your Diet

Embracing the Art of Culinary Diversity:
A Symphony of Flavors for Your Well-Being
Incorporating a diverse array of foods into your diet is not just a culinary delight; it's a celebration of health, vitality, and the rich tapestry of global cuisines. The beauty of variety extends beyond the taste buds, encompassing a spectrum of nutrients, colors, and cultural influences that contribute to your overall well-being. Here's a journey into the

world of culinary diversity, urging you to savor the symphony of flavors that a varied diet can bring to your plate:

1.A Nutrient-Rich Palette:

A wide spectrum of nutrients is ensured via variety. Different foods bring unique combinations of vitamins, minerals, antioxidants, and phytochemicals, providing your body with the diverse nourishment it craves.

2.Exploration of Global Flavors:

Diversify your palate by exploring global cuisines. From the vibrant spices of Indian curries to the umami richness of Japanese sushi,

each culinary tradition adds a unique and enriching dimension to your dining experience.

3. Colorful Culinary Adventure:

A colorful plate is not just visually appealing; it signifies a spectrum of health benefits. The vibrant hues of fruits and vegetables often indicate a variety of antioxidants, promoting cellular health and resilience.

4. Plant-Based Pleasures:

Introduce a medley of plant-based delights into your meals. From the earthy goodness of lentils to the creamy texture of avocados, plant-based options offer a rich tapestry of flavors and nutritional benefits.

5.Seafood Symphony:

Include a variety of seafood to benefit from the unique nutritional profiles of different fish and shellfish. From omega-3 fatty acids in salmon to the lean protein of shrimp, the ocean offers a bounty of healthful options.

6. Wholesome Grains and Pulses:

Explore the world of grains and pulses beyond the familiar. Quinoa, farro, lentils, and chickpeas bring both texture and nutrition, elevating your meals with their distinct tastes and health benefits.

7.Artistry in Culinary Techniques:

Play with diverse culinary techniques to enhance flavors. Grilling, roasting, sautéing, and slow-cooking each impart unique tastes, textures, and aromas to your dishes.

8. Seasonal Sensations:

Embrace the beauty of seasonal produce. The flavors of fruits and vegetables at their peak not only taste better but also provide optimal nutritional value, connecting you to the natural rhythms of the earth.

9. Shared Meals, Shared Stories: Gather with loved ones over diverse meals. Sharing the experience of different cuisines fosters connection, cultural appreciation, and the joy of discovering new culinary treasures together.

Finding Joy in Nourishing Foods

Nourishing your body isn't merely a functional task; it's an opportunity to cultivate joy, gratitude, and a profound connection with the essence of life. When approached with mindfulness and appreciation, every meal becomes a celebration of well-being. Here's a journey into the art of finding joy in nourishing foods, transforming each bite into a moment of pure bliss:

1. Mindful Savoring:
Slow down and savor each bite. Engage your senses in the textures, aromas, and flavors of your meal. Mindful savoring allows you to fully appreciate the culinary symphony that unfolds on your palate.

2. Culinary Creativity: Embrace the creativity of cooking. Whether experimenting with new recipes or adding a personal touch to familiar dishes, the act of creating nourishing meals becomes an expressive and joyful endeavor.

3. Gratitude for Earth's Bounty:

Eat to overcome your diet

Cultivate gratitude for the abundance of nourishing foods provided by the Earth. Recognize the journey from soil to plate, acknowledging the interconnectedness of all living things in the cycle of sustenance.

4. Colors of Happiness: Celebrate the vibrant colors on your plate. The rainbow of fruits and vegetables not only signifies diverse nutrients but also brings a visual feast, elevating the aesthetic pleasure of your meals.

5. Connection to Cultural Heritage:
Explore and honor your cultural heritage through traditional cuisines. Connecting with the flavors and dishes of your roots fosters a sense of identity, continuity, and joy derived from culinary traditions.

7. Shared Meals, Shared Joy:

Eat to overcome your diet

Share nourishing meals with loved ones. The act of breaking bread together fosters a sense of community, joy, and the shared experience of enjoying wholesome, delicious food.

8. Guilt-Free Pleasures:

Allow yourself guilt-free pleasures. Indulging in occasional treats or favorite comfort foods without guilt contributes to a positive relationship with food and enhances the joy derived from eating.

9. Mindful Grains of Gratitude:

Pause before meals to express gratitude. Acknowledge the efforts behind the preparation, the nourishment provided, and the privilege of having access to a variety of foods that contribute to your well-being.

10. Holistic Nourishment:

Understand that nourishment extends beyond physical health. Nourishing foods have the power to uplift your mood, enhance your energy levels, and contribute to a holistic sense of well-being and joy.

CHAPTER 4

Overcoming Diet Challenges

Navigating and Overcoming Diet Challenges: A Path to Sustainable Wellness

Embarking on a journey toward a healthier diet often comes with its share of challenges. However, overcoming these hurdles is a crucial step toward achieving sustainable wellness. Here's a guide to help you navigate and conquer common diet challenges, empowering you to make positive, lasting changes:

1. Setting Realistic Goals:

Start by establishing reasonable and doable objectives. Avoid extreme diets or sudden, drastic changes. Gradual, sustainable adjustments are more likely to become lasting habits.

2. Understanding Triggers:

Identify emotional or situational triggers that lead to unhealthy eating habits. Whether it's stress, boredom, or social occasions, recognizing triggers allows you to develop healthier coping mechanisms.

3. Meal Planning and Preparation:

Plan your meals and prepare in advance. This helps you make mindful choices and reduces

the likelihood of opting for convenient, less nutritious options in moments of hunger or time constraints.

4. Diversifying Your Options:

Eat to overcome your diet

Combat boredom or monotony by diversifying your food choices. Explore new recipes, ingredients, and cooking methods to keep your meals exciting and satisfying.

5.Handling Social Pressures:

Navigate social situations where unhealthy food choices may be prevalent. Communicate your dietary preferences with friends and family, and be prepared with healthier alternatives during gatherings.

6. Mindful Eating Practices:

Practice mindful eating to enhance awareness of hunger and fullness. Slow down, savor each bite, and be present during meals to prevent overeating and promote a healthier relationship with food.

7. Addressing Emotional Eating:

If emotional eating is a challenge, seek alternative ways to cope with emotions, such as exercise, journaling, or talking to a friend. Understanding and addressing the root causes can help break the cycle.

8. Seeking Professional Guidance:

Consider consulting a registered dietitian or nutritionist. Professional guidance can provide personalized advice, tailored to your specific needs and challenges, ensuring a more effective and sustainable approach.

9. Flexibility in Dietary Choices:

Embrace flexibility in your dietary choices. Allow yourself occasional treats or deviations from your plan without guilt. A balanced, forgiving approach is key to long-term success.

10. Staying Hydrated:

Sometimes, feelings of hunger may be a sign of dehydration. Stay hydrated throughout the day, as adequate water intake can support overall well-being and help regulate appetite.

11.Tracking Progress Positively:

Track your progress with a positive mindset. Celebrate small victories, whether they're related to better food choices, increased physical activity, or improved well-being. Positive reinforcement boosts motivation.

12. Cultivating a Support System:

Surround yourself with a supportive community. Share your goals with friends or family members who encourage your journey, providing motivation and accountability.

Eat to overcome your diet

Overcoming diet challenges is a continuous process of self-discovery and resilience. By approaching these challenges with patience, self-compassion, and a commitment to long-term well-being, you can create sustainable habits that contribute to a healthier and more fulfilling life.

Dealing with Cravings

A Holistic Approach to Taming Temptations
Cravings, those irresistible urges for specific foods, can present a challenge on the path to maintaining a balanced and healthy lifestyle. Understanding the nuances of cravings and implementing effective strategies to deal with them can empower you to navigate this aspect of your relationship with food. Here's a comprehensive guide to help you decode

cravings and adopt a holistic approach to managing them:

1. Listen to Your Body:

Pay attention to your body's signals. Cravings can sometimes be your body's way of communicating nutritional needs. If you're craving chocolate, for example, it might indicate a need for magnesium found in dark chocolate.

2. Balanced and Nutrient-Rich Diet:

Ensure your meals are well-balanced and nutrient-dense. A diet rich in whole foods, including fruits, vegetables, lean proteins, and whole grains, can help stabilize blood sugar levels and minimize sudden cravings.

3. Opt for Healthy Alternatives:

Eat to overcome your diet

When a specific craving arises, choose healthier alternatives. If you're craving something sweet, opt for a piece of fruit or a small serving of Greek yogurt with honey. Satisfy the craving with nutrient-dense options.

4. Understand Emotional Triggers:
Identify emotional triggers associated with cravings. Stress, boredom, or specific emotions can contribute to the desire for certain foods. Overcoming emotional cravings may require finding alternate techniques for managing emotions.

5. Portion Management and Mindful Indulgence: Give yourself treats once in a while, but watch how much you eat.

Eat to overcome your diet

Enjoying small amounts of your favorite treat mindfully can satisfy the craving without derailing your overall dietary goals.

6. Regular Physical Activity:

Engage in regular physical activity. Exercise not only contributes to overall well-being but can also help regulate appetite and reduce cravings. Find activities you enjoy to make staying active a pleasurable part of your routine.

7. Sufficient Sleep:

Prioritize adequate sleep. Hormonal balance might be upset and cravings can increase when sleep deprived. Establishing a consistent sleep routine supports overall health and well-being.

8. Mindful Snacking:

Eat to overcome your diet

If snacking is a part of your routine, choose nutritious snacks mindfully. Nuts, seeds, or a small serving of veggies with hummus can be satisfying options that contribute to your nutritional goals.

9. Journaling:

Keep a food journal to track your cravings. Note the circumstances surrounding each craving, including emotions, time of day, and what you ate before. This can offer insightful information on trends and causes.

10. Seek Professional Guidance:

If cravings persist or are challenging to manage, consider seeking guidance from a registered dietitian or nutritionist. A professional can provide personalized advice tailored to your specific needs and goals.

Eat to overcome your diet

Approaching cravings with a holistic mindset involves understanding the interconnectedness of physical, emotional, and lifestyle factors. By incorporating these strategies, you not only address the immediate challenge of cravings but also cultivate a sustainable and mindful relationship with food, ultimately supporting your journey to overall well-being.

Strategies for Dining Out

Savvy Strategies for a Healthier Experience

Dining out can be a delightful experience, filled with tantalizing flavors and social enjoyment. However, it also presents the challenge of navigating menus that may tempt you with less-than-healthy options. With a mindful approach and strategic choices, you can savor the dining-out experience while staying true to your health and wellness goals. Here are savvy

Eat to overcome your diet

strategies to guide you through the culinary landscape when dining out:

1.Preview the Menu in Advance:
Before heading to the restaurant, take a peek at the menu online. This allows you to make informed choices in a relaxed environment, avoiding impulsive decisions influenced by hunger or external factors.

2. Choose Restaurants with Healthier Options:
Opt for restaurants that offer a variety of nutritious choices. Many establishments now include lighter or vegetarian options, making it easier to find a meal that aligns with your health goals.

3. Prioritize Vegetables and Lean Proteins:

Build your meal around vegetables and lean proteins. These components not only provide essential nutrients but also contribute to a satisfying and balanced dining experience.

4. Smart Starters:

Begin with a light and nutrient-packed starter. A salad, broth-based soup, or vegetable-based appetizer can help curb hunger and prevent overindulgence in the main course.

5. Customize Your Order:

Don't hesitate to customize your order. Ask for dressings or sauces on the side, opt for grilled or steamed preparations, and inquire about substitutions to tailor the meal to your preferences.

6. Beware of Liquid Calories:

Eat to overcome your diet

Be cautious with liquid calories. Sugary beverages and alcoholic drinks can contribute to overall calorie intake. Choose water, herbal tea, or sparkling water as alternatives to stay hydrated without excess calories.

7. Share Desserts:
If you have a sweet tooth, consider sharing desserts with your dining companions. This way, you can enjoy a taste without overindulging in a full portion.

8. Practice Mindful Eating:
Slow down and savor each bite. Mindful eating allows you to fully appreciate the flavors and textures of your meal, and it can also help you recognize when you're satisfied, preventing overeating.

Eat to overcome your diet

9 . Stay Active Post-Meal:

Consider incorporating physical activity after your meal. A leisurely stroll can aid digestion and contribute to overall well-being, especially if the dining experience includes indulgent choices.

10. Socialize Without Overeating:

Prioritize the social aspect of dining out without making it solely about the food. Engage in meaningful conversations and enjoy the company of friends or family, placing less emphasis on the act of eating.

11 . Practice Moderation, Not Deprivation:

Strive for balance rather than strict deprivation. Allowing yourself occasional indulgences or treats ensures a more sustainable and enjoyable approach to dining out.

Eat to overcome your diet

Mastering the art of dining out involves making mindful choices that align with your health and wellness goals. By incorporating these strategies, you can relish the culinary experience while nurturing your overall well-being, creating a harmonious balance between enjoyment and health-conscious choices.

Handling Social Pressures

Navigating Social Pressures with Grace: Strategies for Authentic Living
In a world that often emphasizes conformity, handling social pressures with resilience and authenticity is a valuable skill. Whether it's societal expectations, peer influence, or cultural norms, staying true to yourself while navigating social dynamics is essential for maintaining mental and emotional well-being. Here's a guide

to help you handle social pressures with grace and authenticity:

1. Know Your Values:

Establish a clear understanding of your values and priorities. Knowing what matters to you provides a solid foundation for making decisions aligned with your authentic self, even in the face of social pressures.

2. Set Boundaries:

Learn to set healthy boundaries. Communicate your limits assertively and respectfully, letting others know when a situation or request goes against your values or personal comfort.

3. Confidence in Individuality:

Embrace your individuality with confidence. Recognize that each person is unique, and your

Eat to overcome your diet

authenticity contributes to the diversity that makes social interactions rich and meaningful.

4. Practice Self-Reflection:
Regularly engage in self-reflection. Understand your motivations, desires, and fears.
This self-awareness empowers you to make decisions that align with your authentic self rather than succumbing to external pressures.

5.Choose Your Circle Wisely:
Be in the company of encouraging and like-minded people. Choose friends and companions who appreciate and respect your

authenticity, fostering an environment where you can be yourself without judgment.

6. Develop Assertiveness Skills:

Build assertiveness skills to express your thoughts, feelings, and needs effectively. Being assertive allows you to navigate social situations with clarity, ensuring your voice is heard while maintaining respect for others.

7. Cultivate Self-Confidence:

Nurture your self-confidence. Acknowledge your strengths and achievements, and celebrate your unique qualities. A strong sense of self-confidence acts as a shield against external pressures.

8. Resist Comparisons:

Avoid the trap of constant comparison. Recognize that everyone has their own journey, and your path may differ from others. Focus on

Eat to overcome your diet

your growth and accomplishments without measuring them against external standards.

9.Learn to Say No:

 Practice saying no when necessary. It's okay to decline invitations or requests that don't align with your priorities. Learning to say no with tact and firmness is a key aspect of maintaining authenticity.

10. Seek Support:

 Reach out for support when needed. Whether from friends, family, or a mental health professional, having a supportive network can provide guidance and encouragement in navigating social pressures.

11. Embrace Imperfections:

Embrace imperfections as part of being human. Allow yourself room for growth and learning.

Eat to overcome your diet

Accepting your flaws and vulnerabilities contributes to a more authentic and compassionate approach to yourself and others.

12. Cultivate a Sense of Humor:

Develop a sense of humor about life's challenges. The ability to find humor in situations can diffuse tension and lighten the mood, making it easier to navigate social pressures with a lighthearted perspective.

Handling social pressures requires a blend of self-awareness, resilience, and a commitment to living authentically. By incorporating these strategies into your life, you empower yourself to navigate social dynamics with grace, staying true to your values and embracing the richness of your unique journey

CHAPTER 5

Fitness and Wellness

Harmony of Body and Mind: A Comprehensive Guide to Fitness and Wellness.

Achieving optimal well-being involves a holistic approach that encompasses both physical fitness and mental wellness. The interplay between a healthy body and a balanced mind is the foundation for a fulfilling and vibrant life. Here's a comprehensive guide to help you navigate the realms of fitness and wellness, fostering a harmonious connection between your body and mind:

1. Physical Fitness:

Eat to overcome your diet

Physical fitness is the cornerstone of a healthy lifestyle. Incorporate a mix of cardiovascular exercise, strength training, and flexibility exercises into your routine to promote overall fitness.

2. Cardiovascular Exercise:

Engage in activities that elevate your heart rate and improve cardiovascular health. Running, cycling, swimming, or brisk walking are excellent choices to enhance endurance and stamina.

3. Strength Training:

Incorporate strength training activities to develop and tone your muscles. Resistance training, weightlifting, or bodyweight exercises contribute to improved strength, metabolism, and overall functional fitness.

4. Flexibility and Mobility:

Prioritize flexibility and mobility exercises. Stretching, yoga, or Pilates can enhance flexibility, reduce the risk of injuries, and contribute to improved posture and range of motion.

5. Mind-Body Connection:

Recognize the profound connection between physical and mental well-being. Exercise triggers the release of endorphins, which are feel-good and stress-relieving neurotransmitters.

6. Holistic Nutrition:

Nourish your body with a well-balanced and nutritious diet. Emphasize whole foods, including fruits, vegetables, lean proteins, whole grains, and healthy fats, to support overall health and energy levels.

7.Hydration:

Stay adequately hydrated. Water is essential for digestion, nutrient absorption, and maintaining bodily functions. Proper hydration contributes to vibrant skin, joint health, and overall well-being.

8. Quality Sleep:

Prioritize quality sleep. Adequate and restful sleep is crucial for physical recovery, cognitive function, and emotional well-being. Establish a consistent sleep routine for optimal health.

9. Stress Management:

Eat to overcome your diet

Practice stress management techniques. Whether through meditation, deep breathing, or mindfulness, managing stress is vital for mental clarity, emotional balance, and overall resilience.

10. Mindfulness Practices:

Embrace mindfulness practices in daily life. Mindful eating, walking, or simply being present in the moment enhances self-awareness and contributes to a sense of peace and tranquility.

11. Social Connection:

Cultivate social connections. Strong social bonds contribute to emotional well-being. Whether through family, friends, or community activities, social engagement is a vital aspect of overall wellness.

12. Holistic Approach:

Adopt a holistic approach to fitness and wellness. Recognize that the synergy between physical health and mental well-being creates a harmonious and sustainable foundation for a fulfilling life.

13. Regular Health Check-ups:

Schedule regular health check-ups. Routine screenings and assessments can detect potential health issues early, allowing for proactive management and prevention.

14. Lifelong Learning:

Foster a mindset of lifelong learning. Continuously seek knowledge about health, nutrition, and fitness. Staying informed

Eat to overcome your diet

empowers you to make informed choices for your well-being.

15. Celebrate Progress:

Celebrate your fitness and wellness journey. Acknowledge and celebrate your achievements, whether they are physical milestones, mental resilience, or positive lifestyle changes.

Remember, the journey to optimal well-being is a personal and evolving process. By integrating these elements into your life, you pave the way for a harmonious interplay between physical fitness and mental wellness, creating a foundation for a fulfilling and vibrant existence

The Role of Exercise in a Balanced Lifestyle

Elevating Life's Symphony: The Intrinsic Role of Exercise in a Balanced Lifestyle

Exercise is not merely a component of a healthy lifestyle; it's the rhythmic heartbeat that propels the entire symphony of well-being. The profound impact of regular physical activity extends far beyond muscle toning and

cardiovascular health—it permeates every aspect of our lives, contributing to mental clarity, emotional resilience, and a balanced existence. Here's an exploration of the intrinsic role of exercise in creating a harmonious and fulfilling lifestyle:

Eat to overcome your diet

1. Physical Vitality:

Exercise is the engine that fuels physical vitality. Regular activity enhances endurance, strength, and flexibility, laying the foundation for a body that moves with grace and resilience.

2. Cardiovascular Health:

The rhythmic dance of cardiovascular exercise elevates heart health. Activities such as running, cycling, or swimming strengthen the heart,

improving circulation and reducing the risk of cardiovascular diseases.

3. Mental Clarity and Focus:

Exercise is a cognitive elixir. The increased blood flow and oxygen to the brain during physical activity enhance mental clarity, focus, and cognitive function, promoting sharper decision-making and problem-solving skills.

4. Stress Reduction:

Sweating it out on the exercise mat or trail is a powerful stress-buster. Physical activity triggers the release of endorphins, the body's natural stress relievers, creating a soothing balm for the mind.

5. Emotional Well-Being:

The connection between exercise and emotional well-being is profound. Regular physical activity has been linked to reduced symptoms of anxiety and depression, fostering a positive and resilient emotional state.

6. Enhanced Sleep Quality:

The lullaby of exercise contributes to improved sleep quality. A well-rested body and mind, rejuvenated through restorative sleep, are vital components of a balanced and energized lifestyle.

7. Weight Management:

Exercise is a loyal companion on the journey of weight management. Combined with a balanced diet, regular physical activity helps maintain a

healthy weight and supports body composition goals.

8. Improved Immune Function:

The immune system performs a robust symphony when fueled by exercise. Regular moderate-intensity activity has been associated

Eat to overcome your diet

with enhanced immune function, contributing to overall health and resilience against illnesses.

9. Social Connection:
Group exercise or team sports contribute to social connection. The camaraderie and shared goals foster a sense of community, enriching life beyond the physical benefits of the activity.

10. Building Healthy Habits:
Exercise is a cornerstone for building a foundation of healthy habits. The discipline and consistency required in a fitness routine often spill over into other areas of life, creating a ripple effect of positive lifestyle choices.

11. Increased Energy Levels:

Far from depleting energy, exercise is an energy amplifier. The surge of endorphins and improved circulation leave you feeling invigorated, translating into increased energy levels for daily activities.

12. Long-Term Health:

Regular exercise is an investment in long-term health. It contributes to the prevention of chronic conditions, such as diabetes and

osteoporosis, promoting not just longevity but a high quality of life.

13. Mind-Body Harmony:

Exercise bridges the gap between body and mind, fostering a harmonious connection. The holistic benefits contribute to a sense of

Eat to overcome your diet

balance, allowing individuals to navigate the complexities of life with greater ease.

14. Adaptability and Resilience:

The adaptability cultivated through exercise—whether facing physical challenges or pushing personal boundaries—translates into resilience. This mental toughness becomes a valuable asset in navigating life's uncertainties.

15. Enjoyment and Recreation:

Last but not least, exercise is a celebration of movement and recreation. Finding joy in physical activity, whether through dancing, hiking, or playing sports, adds a layer of enjoyment that transforms exercise from a routine into a cherished part of life.

Integrating Physical Activity into Your Routine

Seamless Strides: Integrating Physical Activity into Your Daily Routine

Amid the hustle and bustle of modern life, finding time for physical activity can seem like a challenge. However, weaving movement into your routine doesn't necessarily require a complete overhaul. By embracing a mindset of

integration, you can effortlessly incorporate physical activity into your daily life. Here's a guide on seamlessly infusing movement into your routine for a healthier and more active lifestyle:

1. Start with Small Steps:

Eat to overcome your diet

Begin with small, achievable changes. Opt for the stairs instead of the elevator, take short breaks to stretch, or choose a parking spot farther from your destination. These subtle adjustments lay the foundation for a more active lifestyle.

2. Set Realistic Goals:

Set achievable and realistic goals for physical activity. Whether it's a daily 10-minute walk, a quick home workout, or incorporating active hobbies, having tangible goals makes it easier to integrate movement into your routine.

3. Choose Activities You Enjoy:

Select activities that bring you joy. Whether it's dancing, hiking, cycling, or playing a sport, integrating activities you enjoy increases the likelihood of making them a consistent part of your routine.

4. Make It Social:
Turn physical activity into a social affair. Invite friends or family to join you for a walk, hike, or fitness class. Shared activities not only contribute to your health but also foster social connections.

5. Leverage Breaks at Work:
Use breaks at work to incorporate movement. Stretch, take a short walk, or do simple exercises to break up long periods of sitting. These micro-movements contribute to overall well-being.

6. Multitask Mindfully:

Eat to overcome your diet

Multitask mindfully by incorporating movement into daily chores. While waiting for your coffee to brew, do a few stretches. Turn mundane tasks like vacuuming or gardening into opportunities for physical activity.

7. Explore Active Commuting:

Consider active commuting options. If feasible, walk or bike to work, or use public transportation combined with walking. This not only adds physical activity to your day but also reduces environmental impact.

8. Create a Home Workout Space:

Develop a simple home workout space. Whether it's a corner with a yoga mat, resistance bands, or dumbbells, having a designated area makes it convenient to engage in quick exercises at home.

9. Prioritize Morning Movement:

Kickstart your day with morning movement. Whether it's a short workout, yoga, or a brisk walk , incorporating physical activity in the morning sets a positive tone for the day.

10. Dance to the Beat:

Embrace the joy of dancing. Whether it's in your living room or during daily chores, dancing is a fun and effective way to infuse movement into your routine.

11. Utilize Technology:

Leverage fitness apps or online workouts. With a plethora of resources available, you can access guided workouts that suit your preferences and time constraints, making it easier to integrate physical activity.

12. Schedule Active Breaks:

Integrate active breaks into your schedule. Set reminders to stand up, stretch, or take a short walk at regular intervals throughout the day, ensuring consistent movement.

13. Engage in Active Hobbies:

Explore hobbies that involve physical activity. Whether it's gardening, dancing, or playing a musical instrument, incorporating movement
Into Hobbies and enjoyable dimension to your routine.

14. Track Your Progress:

Use fitness trackers or apps to monitor your daily activity. Tracking progress provides motivation and a tangible way to see how small

Eat to overcome your diet

changes contribute to your overall physical well-being.

15.Celebrate Consistency:

Celebrate your consistent efforts. Recognize that integrating physical activity is an ongoing process, and every small step contributes to a healthier and more active lifestyle.

Achieving Overall Well-Being

Holistic Harmony: Achieving Overall Well-Being

True well-being extends beyond mere physical health; it encompasses the harmonious integration of physical, mental, and emotional facets of our lives. Achieving overall well-being involves nurturing each aspect, creating a

Eat to overcome your diet

holistic tapestry that contributes to a fulfilled and balanced existence. Here's a comprehensive guide to guide you on the journey toward holistic well-being:

1. Cultivate Mindfulness:
Begin by cultivating mindfulness. Be present in the moment, paying attention to your thoughts, feelings, and surroundings.
Mindfulness fosters self-awareness, a crucial foundation for overall well-being.

2. Nourish Your Body:
Prioritize nutrition as a cornerstone of well-being. Embrace a balanced and nutrient-rich diet that includes a variety of

Eat to overcome your diet

fruits, vegetables, whole grains, lean proteins, and healthy fats to support physical health.

3. Regular Physical Activity:
Integrate regular physical activity into your routine. Exercise not only enhances physical health but also contributes to mental clarity, emotional balance, and overall vitality.

4. Quality Sleep:
 Prioritize quality sleep. Establish a consistent sleep routine and create a sleep-conducive environment. Adequate and restful sleep is

essential for physical recovery and mental well-being.

5. Stress Management:

Eat to overcome your diet

Develop effective stress management techniques. Whether through meditation, deep breathing, or engaging in relaxing activities, managing stress is crucial for overall well-being.

6. Cultivate Healthy Relationships:

Foster healthy relationships. Surround yourself with supportive and positive individuals who contribute to your emotional well-being. Cultivating meaningful connections enhances overall life satisfaction.

7. Emotional Intelligence:

Develop emotional intelligence. Understand and navigate your emotions effectively, fostering resilience and the ability to adapt to life's challenges with grace.

8. Continuous Learning:

Cultivate a mindset of continuous learning. Embrace curiosity and seek opportunities for personal and professional growth. Lifelong learning contributes to a sense of purpose and fulfillment.

9. Work-Life Balance:

Strive for a healthy work-life balance. Establish boundaries between work and personal life, ensuring time for relaxation, recreation, and meaningful activities outside of professional responsibilities.

10. Express Creativity:

Engage in creative expression. Whether through art, writing, or other forms of self-expression, creativity adds a vibrant dimension to life and fosters a sense of fulfillment.

11. Connect with Nature

Spend time in nature. Connecting with the natural world has been linked to improved mental health and well-being. Take walks in parks, hike in nature reserves, or simply enjoy outdoor activities.

12. Practice Gratitude:

Cultivate a practice of gratitude. Recognize and value your life's positive features on a regular basis. Gratitude enhances overall well-being by

shifting focus to the positive aspects of your experiences.

13. Set Meaningful Goals:

Set meaningful and achievable goals. Whether personal or professional, having goals provides direction and purpose, contributing to a sense of accomplishment and well-being.

14. Mind-Body Practices:

Incorporate mind-body practices. Yoga, meditation, and tai chi are examples of practices that integrate physical and mental well-being, promoting a holistic approach to overall health.

15. Contribute to Others:

Engage in acts of kindness and contribute to others. Volunteering or supporting your

community fosters a sense of connection and purpose, enriching your overall well-being.

Conclusion

In concluding "Eat to Overcome Your Diet," we find ourselves at the intersection of mindful nutrition and empowered living. This book has transcended conventional dieting paradigms, offering not just a guide to what's on your plate but a holistic approach to transforming your relationship with food. We've delved into the profound impact of balanced nutrition, explored strategies for overcoming diet challenges, and discovered the joy in nourishing foods.

As you embark on the journey beyond diets, remember that this is not a rigid path but a dynamic exploration of self-discovery. The principles shared within these pages aim to empower you to make informed choices, cultivate a positive relationship with food, and achieve sustainable well-being. Embrace the art of mindful eating, savor the diverse flavors of nutrient-rich meals, and relish the freedom of a lifestyle that prioritizes nourishment over restrictive diets.

In every bite, find an opportunity to celebrate the vibrant tapestry of flavors and nutrients that contribute not just to physical health but to a profound sense of vitality. As you navigate the challenges and victories on your journey, may this book serve as a compass, guiding you toward a life where every meal becomes a mindful and joyous affirmation of your commitment to nourishing your body, mind, and spirit. Eat to overcome not just the limitations of diets but to overcome the barriers to a life

Eat to overcome your diet

truly well-lived. Here's to your health, your joy, and your journey beyond diets!